GUIDELINES FOR COMPREHENSIVE PROGRAMS TO PROMOTE HEALTHY EATING AND PHYSICAL ACTIVITY

Nutrition and Physical Activity Work Group

Susanne Gregory, MPH

Editor

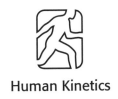

Human Kinetics

Library of Congress Cataloging-in-Publication Data

ISBN: 0-7360-4464-7
Copyright © 2002 by Nutrition and Physical Activity Work Group

Managing Editor: Coree Schutter; **Assistant Editor:** Scott Hawkins; **Copyeditor:** Scott Weckerly; **Graphic Designer:** Stuart Cartwright; **Graphic Artist:** Dawn Sills; **Cover Designer:** Keith Blomberg; **Photographer (interior):** pgs. 1 and 17 courtesy of the California Nutrition Network and California 5 a Day—for Better Health! campaigns; pgs. 7, 11, and 25 © Susanne Phelan Gregory, 2001; page 13 Centers for Disease Control and Prevention; page 21 Tom Roberts; **Printer:** United Graphics

Printed in the United States of America   10   9   8   7   6   5   4

Human Kinetics

Web site: www.HumanKinetics.com

United States: Human Kinetics, P.O. Box 5076, Champaign, IL 61825-5076
800-747-4457
e-mail: humank@hkusa.com

Canada: Human Kinetics, 475 Devonshire Road Unit 100, Windsor, ON N8Y 2L5
800-465-7301 (in Canada only)
e-mail: orders@hkcanada.com

Europe: Human Kinetics, 107 Bradford Road, Stanningley, Leeds LS28 6AT, United Kingdom
+44 (0) 113 255 5665
e-mail: hk@hkeurope.com

Australia: Human Kinetics, 57A Price Avenue, Lower Mitcham, South Australia 5062
08 8277 1555
e-mail: liaw@hkaustralia.com

New Zealand: Human Kinetics, Division of Sports Distributors NZ Ltd., P.O. Box 300 226 Albany, North Shore City, Auckland
0064 9 448 1207
e-mail: blairc@hknewz.com

FOR CO_____IVE
PROGRAMS TO
PROMOTE HEALTHY EATING
AND PHYSICAL ACTIVITY

In memory of those who died on September 11th
and for a nation that must continue—
we dedicate this document to those who work every day
to bring joy and health to our communities.

CONTENTS

Nutrition and Physical Activity Work Group Representatives ix

Preface xi

Acknowledgments xiii

Introduction xv

I. Leadership, Planning/Management, and Coordination 1

II. Environmental, Systems, and Policy Change 7

III. Mass Communication 11

IV. Community Programs and Community Development 13

V. Programs for Children and Youth 17

VI. Health Care Delivery 21

VII. Surveillance, Epidemiology, and Research 25

Appendix A   Funding Case Studies for Nutrition and Physical Activity Programs 29

Appendix B   Linking the Guidelines to the Essential Public Health Services 37

NUTRITION AND PHYSICAL ACTIVITY WORK GROUP REPRESENTATIVES

Association of State and Territorial Chronic Disease Program Directors

- Don Bishop, PhD, Chief of Center for Health Promotion, Minnesota Department of Health
- Jack Hataway, MD, MPH, Director of Chronic Disease Prevention Division, Bureau of Health Promotion and Information, Alabama Department of Public Health

Association of State and Territorial Directors of Health Promotion and Public Health Education

- Jane M. Moore, PhD, RD, Program Manager for Oregon Department of Human Resources, Chronic Disease Prevention
- Donna C. Nichols, MSEd, CHES, Director of Public Health Promotion, Texas Department of Health

Association of State and Territorial Public Health Nutrition Directors

- Kristin V. Biskeborn, MPH, RD, LN, State Nutritionist Health and Medical Services, South Dakota Department of Health
- Karen J. Oby, MPH, LRD, MCH/WIC Nutrition Services Director of MCH Division, North Dakota Department of Health

National Association for Health and Fitness

- Mike Feulner, Vermont Governor's Council on Physical Fitness and Sports

National Association of City and County Health Officials

- Michael Meit, Director of Community Health Office

National Association of WIC Directors

- Joanne White, RD, Delaware WIC Program

National Public Health Information Coalition

- Mari-jean Siehl, former president of NPHIC, Director of Public Affairs, Ohio Department of Health

Society of State Directors of Health, Physical Education and Recreation

- William H. Datema, MS, Executive Director

State Health Department Representatives (At Large)

- Susan B. Foerster, MPH, RD, Chief of Cancer Prevention and Nutrition Section, California Department of Health Services
- Larry R. Prohs, Ohio Department of Health
- Jeff Sunderlin, Public Health Administrator, Office of Health Promotion, Illinois Department of Public Health
- Sue Wilson, MS, RD, Nutrition Program Manager of WIC and Nutrition Services, Florida Department of Health

United States Department of Agriculture

- Judy Wilson, RD, MSPH, Director of Nutrition Services Staff Office of Analysis, Nutrition and Evaluation, Food and Nutrition Service

PREFACE

Many people in America today die or are disabled by chronic diseases, diseases that could be controlled or even avoided through better nutrition and increased physical activity. Yet making these choices is difficult. As Americans, we live in a society that makes it easy to eat a lot of high-calorie foods and to avoid being active. How can we counteract these trends to make it easier for people to live healthier lifestyles? Our objective in this document is to answer this question.

We are the state Nutrition and Physical Activity Work Group (NUPAWG), and we decided to begin by formulating guidelines for state and local health advocates who want to create their own comprehensive nutrition, physical activity, and obesity control programs. Our group represents key national, state, and local public health and education partners, working together to improve the nation's dietary and physical activity practices. With assistance from the Centers for Disease Control and Prevention's Division of Nutrition and Physical Activity (CDC-DNPA), we developed this document, *Guidelines for Comprehensive Programs to Promote Healthy Eating and Physical Activity*. We used the *Best Practices for Comprehensive Tobacco Control Programs* (1999) as a model for these guidelines.

For this document, we have identified seven program components:

I. Leadership, Planning/Management, and Coordination

II. Environmental, Systems, and Policy Change

III. Mass Communication

IV. Community Programs and Community Development

V. Programs for Children and Youth

VI. Health Care Delivery

VII. Surveillance, Epidemiology, and Research

For each component, we have a rationale for its inclusion, sample activities, sample practices and programs, and resources and references. When choosing practices and programs to include in this document, we looked for those that were

- focused on the elimination of disparities,
- affordable and sustainable,
- population-based,
- science-based and effective,
- replicable and relatively easy to implement,
- well-defined with clear goals and measurable objectives,
- valued by stakeholders,
- comprehensive and inclusive,
- acceptable to the target population,
- accessible, and
- focused on growing communities and building social capital.

Please note that for some activities and examples not all criteria were appropriate.

We are aware that many of the existing nutrition and physical activity programs, policies, and interventions have limited evaluation and data on effectiveness in changing behaviors and improving health outcomes. However, we felt it was important to take a first step toward defining the scope and nature of comprehensive programs for nutrition and physical activity and to highlight examples of programs and interventions that seem to be succeeding. This document captures a point in time, describing the current efforts that address the disease risk factors of suboptimal nutrition and inactivity.

We also have included two appendixes in this document. One describes two case studies about state funding to provide a real-world basis for estimating the funding required to build a statewide comprehensive program. The other links the guidelines in this document to the Essential Public Health Services (EPHS), which are described in the introduction. We created this document to be used with other key public health and chronic disease prevention documents, including the *Healthy People 2010: Objectives for the Nation* (2000), the *CDC Guide to Community Preventive Services* (**http://www.thecommunityguide.org**), and the *CDC Guide to Best Practices in Chronic Disease Prevention and Control* (in press).

We hope this document helps a wide range of people: health department managers, boards of health, voluntary agencies, school administrators, business managers, university research programs, local government and community planners, legislators, advocates, and the media. We think that it is a good start in encouraging the necessary change in American communities that will ultimately result in healthier lives for all.

ACKNOWLEDGMENTS

The members of the Nutrition and Physical Activity Work Group prepared this publication with assistance from staff members at the Centers for Disease Control and Prevention, National Center for Chronic Disease Prevention and Health Promotion, Division of Nutrition and Physical Activity.

INTRODUCTION

Poor diet and physical inactivity cause 310,000 to 580,000 deaths each year and are major contributors to disabilities that result from diabetes, osteoporosis, obesity, and stroke. The facts are clear: We are faced with urgent health issues and startling trends that must be addressed. Consider the following:

- Chronic diseases account for 7 out of every 10 deaths in the United States and for more than 60% of total medical care expenditures.

- Approximately one-third of cancer cases are attributed to poor diet and lack of exercise, the same as the proportion of cancer deaths attributed to smoking.

- For cases of heart disease and hypertension, 20% to 40% are attributed to diet and as much as 90% of diabetes cases may be due to overweight and obesity.

- Approximately 61% of adults are overweight or obese.

- The prevalence of overweight children and adolescents has more than doubled in the last 20 years. At least 10% of school-aged children and 14% of teens are overweight.

- Of the 5- to 10-year-old children that are overweight, 60% have at least one associated biochemical or clinical cardiovascular risk factor such as hyperlipidemia, elevated blood pressure, or increased insulin level.

According to the report *Healthy People 2010* (2000), about 75% of Americans eat too little fruit, 95% eat too few vegetables, and 64% eat too much saturated fat. In addition, 12% of households are food insecure. The diets of many population subgroups exceed recommendations for diet elements such as total fat, saturated fat, and calories, and their diets fall significantly short of the recommendations on other important elements such as calcium for adolescent girls.

Just one in four adults gets sufficient regular physical activity to provide health benefits; another one in four reports no regular physical activity at all. In effect, 60% of American adults do not get the recommended amount of daily physical activity (Healthy People 2010). The trend is not promising for our youths: Physical activity rates drop off sharply in junior high school for girls and in high school for boys. By the end of high school, rates for girls and boys are comparable to adult rates.

Obesity is recognized as the first chronic disease whose spread looks like an infectious disease epidemic. It substantially raises the risk of hypertension, blood cholesterol, type 2 diabetes, coronary heart disease, stroke, gallbladder disease, osteoarthritis, sleep apnea and respiratory problems, and cancers of the endometrium, breast, prostate, and colon. Results from the Third National Health and Nutrition Examination Survey (NHANES III), show that persons with a body mass index (BMI) greater than or equal to 27 have a greater than 70% chance of having an obesity-related comorbidity.

The rapid increase in the prevalence of obesity in the United States is a result of environmental and behavioral factors that foster eating more higher-calorie foods more frequently and burning fewer calories through physical activity. Obesity and a sedentary lifestyle present a serious and growing concern and financial burden for individuals, our health care system, and society.

Obesity is not only an issue for adults. Type 2 diabetes, formerly considered a disease of middle age, is increasing in children and young adults. Recent research indicates that not only do young children have risk factors associated with cardiovascular disease, but atherosclerosis is occurring in preschool children as well.

The chronic disease epidemic takes a disproportionate toll in poor and underserved populations, and the nation has failed in its efforts to reduce chronic disease mortality among these populations. Prevalence and risk of chronic diseases, including the rate of diabetes, stroke, heart disease, being overweight, and obesity, are consistently higher for many populations. For example, while cancer rates for White adults have remained relatively stable during the past 25 years, rates among Black males have increased by 18% and among Black females by nearly 10% (NCHS 1997). The disparity in overall mortality and chronic disease between higher and lower socioeconomic groups continues to increase in the United States (Pappas 1993).

The United States spends more on health care than any nation in the world, yet it continues to have some of the poorest health outcomes in the industrialized world. In part, this disparity is due to an overemphasis on treatment, technology, and health services rather than primary prevention and action to improve social conditions and reduce inequities that cause ill health. Current funding for health promotion programs is limited.

The CDC's Division of Nutrition and Physical Activity has an annual budget of $16 million compared to the $100 million that CDC is given for programs to reduce the use of tobacco, which kills about the same number of Americans as unhealthy eating and physical inactivity. According to the U.S. Department of Agriculture and the CDC, better nutrition and physical activity could reduce health and other costs by at least $148 billion a year.

GOALS OF A COMPREHENSIVE NUTRITION AND PHYSICAL ACTIVITY PROGRAM

The goals of a comprehensive approach to nutrition and physical activity are to

- promote healthy eating that follows national dietary guidance policy;
- maintain recommended levels of moderate and vigorous physical activity from

childhood through adolescence into adulthood;

- eliminate disparities in diet, physical activity, and overweight among disadvantaged population groups;
- increase access to healthy foods and to opportunities to be active for every age and population group; and
- promote healthy weight among adults and children.

The goals and the guidelines outlined in this document are consistent with the focus of the Essential Public Health Services (EPHS) that state that governmental public health agencies serve as facilitating points for assessing performance of EPHS within state or community public health systems. A wide variety of public, private, and voluntary organizations make up a public health system and contribute to EPHS delivery. Coordination of EPHS provides the foundation needed by public health systems to effectively carry out any public health improvement program in states or communities (see appendix B).

Essential Public Health Services

Monitor health status to identify health problems.

Diagnose and investigate health problems and health hazards.

Inform, educate, and empower people about health issues.

Mobilize partnerships to identify and solve health problems.

Develop policies and plans that support individual and statewide health efforts.

Enforce laws and regulations that protect health and ensure safety.

Link people to needed personal health services and ensure the provision of health care when otherwise unavailable.

Ensure a competent public and personal health care **workforce**.

Evaluate effectiveness, accessibility, and quality of personal and population-based health services.

Research new insights and innovative solutions to health problems.

THEORETICAL MODEL

The foundation for these guidelines is based on the understanding that health promotion includes not only educational activities but also advocacy, organizational change efforts, policy development, economic supports, environmental change, and multimethod strategies (*Theory at a Glance*). This ecological perspective highlights the importance of approaching public health problems at multiple levels and stressing interaction and integration of factors within and across levels. When developing this document, NUPAWG members used the social-ecological model as a guide, which has five successively more complex levels (or spheres) of influence:

• **Intrapersonal or individual factors**—Individual characteristics that influence behavior such as knowledge, attitudes, beliefs, and personality traits.

• **Interpersonal factors**—Interpersonal processes and primary groups that include family, friends, and peers, all of which provide social identity, support, and role definition.

• **Institutional factors**—Rules, regulations, policies, and informal structures, which may constrain or promote recommended behaviors.

• **Community factors**—Social networks and norms (or standards), which exist formally or informally among individuals, groups, and organizations.

• **Public policy**—Local, state, and federal policies and laws that regulate or support healthy actions and practices for disease prevention, early detection, control, and management.

A Social-Ecological Model for Levels of Influence

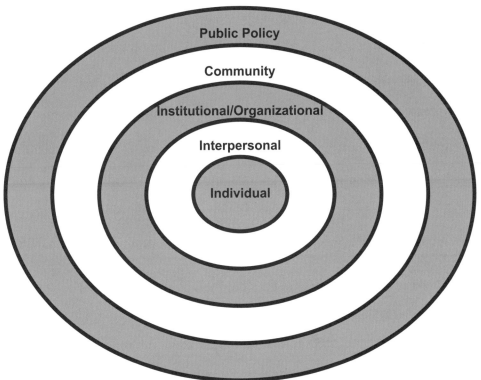

Public Policy: local, state, and federal government policies, regulations, and laws

Community: social networks, norms, standards and practices among organizations

Institutional/Organizational: rules, policies, procedures, environment, and informal structures within an organization or system

Interpersonal: family, friends, peers that provide social identity, support and identity

Individual: awareness, knowledge, attitudes, beliefs, values, preferences

Based on data from McElroy KR, Bibeau D, Steckler A, Glanz K. An ecological perspective on health promotion programs. Health Education Quarterly 15:351-377, 1988.

Research has shown that health promotion succeeds most when promoters analyze problems and plan programs while keeping in mind these various levels of influence. Thus, a comprehensive planning system, such as social marketing, starts with extensive research to assess needs at multiple levels. This research involves consumer and market analysis; epidemiological assessment; behavioral, educational, environmental, and organizational diagnosis; and administrative and policy assessment.

While individual-based intervention programs have been widely used to address nutrition and physical activity, there is a great need to design, implement, and evaluate interventions focused on institutional, community, and policy levels to effect change among large populations.

REFERENCES AND RESOURCES

1. Wolf, AM, Colditz, GA. Current Estimates of the Economic Cost of Obesity in the United States. Obesity Research, 1998; 6(2): 97-106.
2. Pratt M, Macera C, Wang G. Higher Direct Medical Costs Associated with Physical Inactivity. The Physician and Sportsmedicine, 2000; 28(10).
3. Smedley, BD, Syme, SL. Promoting Health: Intervention Strategies from Social and Behavioral Research. Institute of Medicine, 2000.
4. Health and Behavior: The Interplay of Biological Behavioral, and Societal Influences. IOM, 2001.
5. Aim for a Healthy Weight. National Heart, Lung, and Blood Institute. Health Action e-Bulletin, March 2001.
6. Subar, AF, Heimendinger, J, Patterson, BH, Krebs-Smith, SM, Pivonka, E, Kessler, R. Fruit and Vegetable Intake in the United States: The Baseline Survey of the Five-a-Day for Better Health Program. American Journal of Health Promotion, 1995; 9(5): 352-360.
7. Koplan, JP, Dietz, WH. Caloric Imbalance and Public Health Policy. Journal of the American Medical Association, 1999; 282(16): 1579-1581.
8. Mokdad, AH, Serdula, MK, Dietz, WH, Bowman, BA, Marks, JS, Koplan, JP. The Spread of the Obesity Epidemic in the United States, 1991-1998. Journal of the American Medical Association, 1999; 282(16): 1519-1522.
9. Third Report on Nutrition Monitoring in the United States, Interagency Board for Nutrition Monitoring and Related Research, Executive Summary. US Government Printing Office, Washington, DC, December 1995.
10. Nutrition and Your Health: Dietary Guidelines for Americans, Superintendent of Documents, Washington, DC, 2000. ISBN 0-16-050376-0.
11. Best Practices for Comprehensive Tobacco Control Programs—August 1999. CDC, 1999.
12. Physical Activity and Good Nutrition: Essential Elements for Good Health (At-a-Glance). CDC, 1999.
13. Gottlieb, NH, McElroy, KR. Social Health. In Health Promotion in the Workplace. 2nd edition. Eds. M.P. O'Donnell and J.S. Harris. Albany, NY: Delmar Publishers, 1994.
14. Theory-at-a-Glance: A Guide for Health Practitioners. National Institutes of Health, National Cancer Institute, 1995.
15. McGinnis, JM, Foege, WH. Actual Causes of Death in the United States, Journal of the American Medical Association, 1993, Nov 10; 270(18): 2207-2212.
16. Healthy People 2010, Volume II. U.S. Department of Health and Human Services, Washington, DC, January 2000.
17. Zasa S, et al. Scope and Organization of the Guide to Community Preventive Services. The Task Force on Community Prevention Services. American Journal of Preventive Medicine, January 2000; 18(Suppl): 27-34.
18. Fagot-Campagna, A, et al. Type 2 Diabetes among North American Children and Adolescents: An Epidemiological Review and a Public Health Perspective. Journal of Pediatrics, 2000 May; 136(5): 664-672.
19. Berenson, GS, et al. Association between Multiple Cardiovascular Risk Factors and Atherosclerosis in Children and Young Adults. New England Journal of Medicine, 1998, Jun 4; 338: 1650-1656.
20. Pappas G, Queen S, Hadden W, Fisher G. The Increase Disparity in Mortality between Socioeconomic Groups in the United States, 1960 and 1986. New England Journal of Medicine, 1993, Jul 8; 329(2): 103-109.

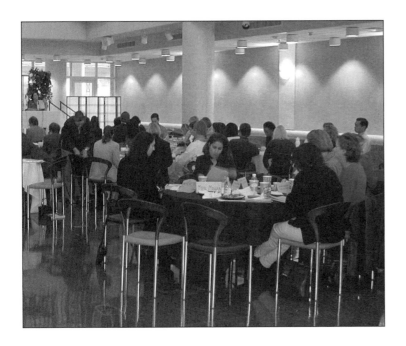

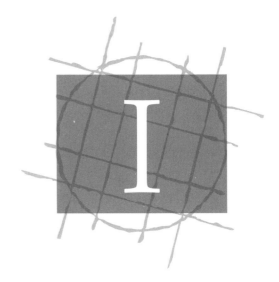

Leadership, Planning/Management, and Coordination

One major obstacle to program effectiveness is a lack of consistency in the delivery of program messages and activities. Therefore, effective first steps in program development are to locate committed leaders, involve all related agencies, and conduct thorough planning so that efforts are coordinated and adequately supported and evaluated. By taking these steps, we can secure funding from multiple streams, use that funding more efficiently, and have a better chance of affecting the target population.

RATIONALE

Three elements are critical for establishing an entity, focus, and vision for nutrition and physical activity: leadership, planning/management, and coordination. Each is discussed in the following sections.

LEADERSHIP

Collective action is required at the federal, state, and local levels to create programs, policies, and practices that encourage healthy eating and physically active lifestyles. Partners at all levels are needed to assume leadership roles in responding to this public health challenge. Elected individuals, employers, community representatives, and school officials must advocate for an environment that makes physical activity and healthy food choices easy, enjoyable, affordable, and safe. Health care dollars are needed to fund prevention. The money needs to be utilized both within health care delivery and within programs in the community.

Each state needs the capacity to frame the issues, create a vision, set goals and objectives, determine strengths, and integrate intervention programs. Along with the visionary elements of leadership comes the crucial need to develop infrastructure and attract resources.

PLANNING/MANAGEMENT

An effective nutrition, physical activity, and obesity prevention program requires strong management structure and planning. Program components must be coordinated, have adequate fiscal and program monitoring, and include effective communication. Management and resource development are cornerstones for effective planning. Leaders who achieve effective planning and management are those who are willing to accept many roles, including convener, facilitator, participant, collaborator/partner, trainer, broker, negotiator, and funder.

COORDINATION

The responsibility for state nutrition and physical activity programs, policy, and practices is spread across state agencies and varies from state to state. At times, messages and methods are disjointed, uncoordinated, and contradictory. In most states, the Department of Education directs the U.S. Department of Agriculture's (USDA) school nutrition programs, such as the National School Lunch Program (NSLP), the Child and Adult Care Feeding Program (CACFP), Team Nutrition, and the School Milk Program (SMP). Education or social service departments may administer the Head Start Program and set the standards for physical education and health curriculums.

Human services departments usually administer the USDA Food Stamp Program, and nutrition programs for the elderly may be administered through an agency for the aging. Medicaid, state children's health insurance programs, and Early and Periodic Screening, Diagnosis, and Treatment (EPSDT) may be administered through the Department of Human Services or the State Health Department, depending on the state. Nutrition services are also provided through Cooperative Extension.

Within state health departments, nutrition and physical activity services are often fragmented: maternal and child health funding and the women, infants, and children (WIC) programs address the needs of children and young families; chronic disease programs ad-

dress several populations with established risk factors; and diabetes programs only recently have started to address primary prevention. Councils on physical fitness may report directly to the governor's office, and little collaboration may exist between departments of parks and recreation or between transportation agencies and health-related agencies and programs.

It is essential that nutrition and physical activity programming be integrated with other programs at the national, state, county, and community levels to achieve the greatest impact for the funding available. The more that consistent eating and physical activity messages are reinforced across programs, the greater chance the consumer will implement a behavior change.

State health departments and other state agencies may sponsor a variety of programs in which physical activity, diet, and obesity prevention and treatment are good practice. These programs include the following:

cardiovascular disease

cancer prevention

diabetes

youth tobacco control

adolescent health programs

school nutrition programs

maternal and child programs

Early and Periodic Screening, Diagnosis, and Treatment (EPSDT)

Special Supplemental Nutrition Program for Women, Infants, and Children (WIC)

Food Stamp Nutrition Education Programs

Social Marketing Networks

5-a-Day Programs

arthritis

obesity prevention

coordinated school health

family planning programs

school health and physical education programs

Other programs, including state-specific health initiatives for women, men, or the elderly

Achieving leadership and focus for nutrition and physical activity can be accomplished in several ways. Perhaps the most successful would be to form a distinct unit or team to develop policies, to provide a primary voice, and to nurture cross-program work that pulls from the expertise and resources of categorical programs. The effect would be a broader, more comprehensive approach to the population, thereby increasing the impact of programs aimed at specific diseases and target populations.

SAMPLE ACTIVITIES

Leadership

1. Identify a core entity or unit to link all other programs with nutrition and physical activity components. Identify organizational placement of the program primarily within nutrition and physical activity. Links for consistent and coordinated communication among all relevant programs should be clear to allow for crosscutting coordination.

2. Focus resources for interventions in communities and populations at greater risk. Design interventions through a community-based process that incorporates the needs and wants of the community.

3. Incorporate supportive policies, programs, and actions within state programs. Work for changes in state rules or policies that affect nutrition and physical activity messages and intervention.

4. Establish statewide partnerships that plan and direct large-scale interventions as well as advocate the implementation and enforcement of legislation and policies that promote physical activity and healthy eating.

5. Assist state and local partners in identifying financial resources for implementing and evaluating program activities.

6. Identify infrastructure and staffing needs to implement population-based strategies to address nutrition and physical activity.

Planning/Management

1. Identify, hire, and supervise key staff with appropriate competencies to plan and implement programs. If these staff members are not employed on staff, the services of consultants, subcontractors, and vendors are required. These include marketing and public relations, as well as media and communications that include media advocacy, creative services, applied evaluation, public health law, resource development, and grant writing. Staffing patterns should include program skills and expertise in the following areas:

- Data collection, management, and analysis
- Epidemiology and surveillance
- Research and evaluation
- Health promotion, education, and communication
- Partnership and coalition building
- Science of physical activity, nutrition, and obesity
- Program coordination, management, and strategic planning
- Social marketing and behavioral science
- Population-based interventions and social and environmental change
- Policy
- Administration and management

2. Monitor, evaluate, and develop strategies to assure the availability, effectiveness, and quality of the personnel needed for the delivery of both personal and population-based services. Develop personnel standards based on *Personnel in Public Health Nutrition in the 1990s* (1995) and the American College of Sports Medicine Certification Standards.

3. Administer funds from multiple sources—for example, state general funds, state special funds (snack and soda taxes, tobacco settlement, fees), grants and contracts from different programs of the federal government, sister state agencies, charitable foundations, and other sources such as direct contributions and the sale of program materials.

4. Assess, analyze, interpret, and disseminate data related to nutrition and physical activity. Assessment activities should include the following: monitoring morbidity and mortality; evaluating socioeconomic factors, risk behavior, and the economic burden associated with poor nutrition and sedentary behaviors; monitoring the environmental and socioeconomic data that affect nutrition and physical activity behaviors; tracking policy and legisla-

tion; and evaluating environmental interventions.

5. Develop and maintain a nutrition and physical activity state plan that includes primary strategies for prevention across state-level programs.

6. Develop a process to determine priority populations for interventions; define the criteria for selecting priority populations in the state; and establish the objectives of the interventions, such as the reduction of racial and ethnic disparities. Both epidemiological and market research information are needed to identify priority populations.

7. Develop methods and systems for local and state program use in evaluating an intervention's effectiveness. These data should be comparable across programs. Efforts should focus on assessing disease burden and risk behavior prevalence at the local level.

8. Establish measures to maintain standards, assure accountability, and monitor programs.

9. Support training for partners and stakeholders (internal and external) that focuses on the attitudes, skills, and key actions to promote population-based interventions for nutrition and physical activity.

Coordination

1. Maximize use of state-level resources through formal interagency memoranda of agreement and through regular meetings with state and local agency staff.

2. Ensure that programs address nutrition and physical activity issues in similar or compatible ways both within programs and in messages to the public.

3. Collaborate with other agencies, voluntary and professional organizations, relevant academic organizations, and the health care industry to share materials and methods for educating health care providers.

4. Assist local health departments and organizations to deliver community-based programs for promoting physical activity and healthy eating by providing technical assistance, training, and funds.

5. Assist local health departments by providing coordinated, timely, and accurate information to the public on nutrition and physical activity; by being proactive with health information; and by working closely with the media.

6. Collaborate with federal agencies on data analysis, coordinated technical assistance, financial support, national nutrition and physical activity promotion campaigns, materials and methods development and training, and state-based surveillance of nutrition and physical activity indicators.

7. Form public and private partnerships to combine intervention strategies and to deliver consistent messages across programs and throughout a community. Partners include government, health and consumer organizations, voluntary organizations, trade organizations, affinity organizations (churches, Kiwanis, service groups), private sector agriculture, food production, marketing, food service, grocery stores, physical activity equipment companies, and transportation agencies.

Sample Practices and Programs

The Healthy Hawaii Initiative—development of a noncategorical approach to blending nutrition, physical activity, and tobacco programs. Strategic planning for environmental and policy related initiatives. Funded by tobacco settlement funds. Support for school-based programs, community grants, a single point of access data warehouse, and professional and public education. **Contact:** Susan Jackson, **sjjackso@mail.health.hi.us**, 808-586-4530.

Virginia Chronic Disease Prevention Program (CDPP)—a coalition of programs at the state and local levels that focus on multiple settings and strategies for chronic disease reduction. Infrastructure has been modified to encourage a comprehensive approach to address chronic disease issues, including collaboration with WIC. Physical activity and nutrition are considered common crosscutting factors for collaboration, communication, and sharing resources. **Contact:** Ramona Schaeffer, **rschaeffer@vdh.state.va.us**, 804-786-5420.

California Cancer Prevention and Nutrition Section—social marketing partnerships with businesses, government entities, nonprofit organizations, and individuals that provide financial and technical assistance for a variety of campaigns for promotion of nutrition and physical activity to food-stamp and low-income households. **Contact:** California Nutrition Network, 916-323-0594.

REFERENCES AND RESOURCES

1. U.S. Department of Health and Human Services, Public Health Services, Centers for Disease Control and Prevention, National Center for Chronic Disease Prevention and Health Promotion, Division of Nutrition and Physical Activity. *Promoting Physical Activity: A Guide for Community Action.* Champaign, IL: Human Kinetics, 1999.

2. Personnel in Public Health Nutrition for the 1990s: A Comprehensive Guide. Eds. Janice M. Dodds, EdD, RD and Mildred Kaufman, MS, RD. August 1991. Available from the Public Health Foundation.

3. American Journal of Preventive Medicine, Theme Issue: Physical Activity Interventions, Volume 15, Number 4, November 1998.

4. Morbidity and Mortality Weekly Report, Guidelines for School Health Programs to Promote Lifelong Healthy Eating, Volume 45, Number RR-9, June 1996.

5. Baranowski, T, Stables, G. Learning What Works and How: Process Evaluation of the 5-a-Day Projects. Health Education and Behavior 2000; 27(2).

6. Frazao, E. The American Diet: Health and Economic Consequences. An Economic Research Service Report. United States Department of Agriculture. Agriculture Information Bulletin Number 711, 1995.

7. Overweight and Obesity Activities. Food and Nutrition Service, USDA. (Handout) 2001.

8. Farris, R, Sanders, C, Stockmyer, C. WISEWOMAN: Reducing Health Disparities in Women. The Digest. Winter 2001: 1, 3-5.

9. Association of State and Territorial Public Health Nutrition Directors and Sarah Pierce. Nutrition and Physical Activity Working Group: Needs Assessment of States. 1999: 33 pp.

10. Summary Report of Listening Session. Toward a National Action Plan on Overweight and Obesity: The Surgeon General's Initiative. Bethesda, Maryland, December 7-8, 2000.

11. Rhein, M, Lafronza, V, Bhandari E, Hawes, J, Hofrichter, R. Advancing Community Public Health Systems in the 21st Century: Emerging Strategies and Innovations from the Turning Point Experience. NACCHO, 2001.

12. Alcala, R, Bell, R. Promoting Nutrition and Physical Activity through Social Marketing: Current Practices and Recommendations. Center for Advanced Studies in Nutrition and Social Marketing, University of California, Davis, June 2000.

13. Unrealized Prevention Opportunities: Reducing the Health and Economic Burden of Chronic Disease. A Report of the National Center for Chronic Disease Prevention and Health Promotion. CDC, March 1997.

14. Pate, et al. Physical Activity and Public Health. A Recommendation for the Centers for Disease Control and Prevention and the American College of Sports Medicine. Journal of the American Medical Association, 1995 Feb 1; 273(5): 402-407.

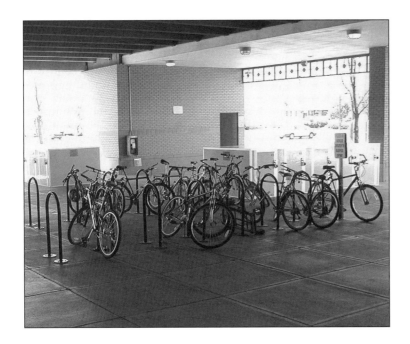

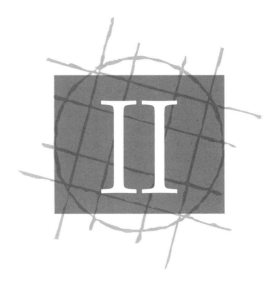

Environmental, Systems, and Policy Change

Although ultimately it is individuals who must change their behavior, many barriers to that change exist in their environments. When we remove those barriers, either by providing circumstances in which good nutrition or physical activity choices are easier to make or by offering incentives for such choices, we support people's personal efforts to change.

RATIONALE

To prevent disease, we ask people to do things that they have not previously done, to stop doing things they have been doing for years, and to do more of some things and less of other things. It is unreasonable to expect that people will change their behaviors easily when so many forces in the social, cultural, and physical environment conspire against such change. If successful programs are to be developed to prevent disease and improve health, then attention must be given not only to the behavior of the people but also to the environment in which they live.

Interventions are most effective when strategies that address individual-level change are (a) implemented concurrently with changes in environments, systems, and policies at the family, community, organization, and societal levels and (b) delivered through a variety of settings.

Intervention efforts should address not only "downstream" individual-level phenomena (e.g., physiologic pathways to disease, individual and lifestyle factors) and "midstream" factors (e.g., population-based interventions), but also "upstream" societal-level phenomena (e.g., public policies).

To create environments, systems, and policies that promote and support behavioral change, we must do the following:

- Eliminate barriers to physical activity—for example, ensure safe, well-maintained recreational areas or support opportunities for physical activity breaks during the workday.
- Eliminate barriers to healthy eating by offering appealing, low-cost fruit and vegetable choices in cafeterias or vending machines.
- Provide explicit support, reinforcement, and inducements for those who make healthy changes or those who are contemplating change.
- Increase resource allocation to areas and populations with greater need (i.e., ensure equitable access to resources for nutrition and physical activity in disadvantaged communities and populations at greater risk for chronic diseases).
- Allocate resources and design policy, environment, and systems strategies for physical activity and nutrition into overall program and chronic disease prevention plans.
- Place emphasis on policy strategies that have broad and sustainable impact across populations and communities.

SAMPLE ACTIVITIES

1. Initiate policy and environmental support in various public places to promote improved nutrition and regular physical activity. Consider the following examples:

- Provide and competitively price nutrient-dense, low-calorie foods in schools, worksites, restaurants, and other food service outlets.
- Alter the choices in food and beverage vending machines to increase the proportion of nutrient-dense, low-calorie foods, such as fruits and vegetables.
- Establish after-hours access to schools for community members to use for indoor recreation.
- Promote stairwell use instead of elevators in the workplace.
- Pass legislation or policy requiring daily physical activity for grades K-12.

2. Promote healthful food advertising and the availability of healthful food, especially in children's environments.

3. Design transportation infrastructure and public policy that supports active modes of transportation, such as walking and biking for both utilitarian and recreational purposes.

4. Form partnerships to ensure that recreation areas and playgrounds in all neighborhoods are safe and in working repair.

Sample Practices and Programs

Safe Routes to School—This California legislation became effective in 2000 and is operated under the Department of Transportation. Projects include installation of sidewalks, crosswalks, bikeways, curbs and gutters, traffic signals, safety lighting, pavement marking, signage, and other improvements to enhance pedestrian and bicycle safety and access near or en route to schools. **Contact:** California Department of Transportation, **www.dot.ca.gov/hq/LocalPrograms/saferoute.htm**.

California Senate Bill 19 (2001)—This limits high-fat and high-sugar-content food and drink in schools. This historic movement exemplified the process of moving legislation forward with community support. The legislation, however, suffered from compromises to child health, but the process is still the best lesson. **Contact:** Harold Goldstein, **HG@PublicHealthAdvocacy.org**, 530-297-6000.

Kids Walk to School—The Walkable South Carolina Committee awarded small grants to 58 schools to promote environmental and policy changes that make walking and bicycling a year-round activity for everyone. Each school uses the *Kids Walk to School* guide to address problems that make walking to school difficult or unsafe. **Contact:** University of South Carolina Prevention Center, **www.prevention.sph.sc.edu**.

Families in Good Health Program—Promotion of physical activity and healthy eating among sedentary residents of Cambodian, Hmong, and Lao communities in Long Beach, California. Barriers to access for fitness were eliminated through collaboration with city government, police, the YMCA, the California Pool for the Handicapped, Buddhist temples, and many other local resources. **Contact:** Southeast Asian Health Project, 310-491-9100.

City of Portland "Reclaiming our Streets"— This project encourages neighborhood livability, alternative transportation, traffic safety, and responsible driver behavior through a traffic-calming program. The Portland Office of Transportation works with neighborhood residents in planning and education efforts. A variety of solutions are used to mitigate the impacts of automobile traffic on neighborhood streets. **Contact:** Transportation Systems Management

Portland Office of Transportation, **www.trans.ci.portland.or.us/Traffic_ Management/Trafficcalming/Default.htm**, 503-823-5185.

TV-Turnoff Network—Emphasizes reduction of television viewing by children and adults. Sponsors a national "TV Turnoff Week" annually with suggestions for alternative activities. Also offers a six-week "More Reading, Less TV" program to encourage children to read instead of watch television. **Contact:** TV-Turnoff Network, **email@TVturnoff.org**, 202-518-5556.

10,000 Steps—This project, developed through a social marketing approach, uses prompts and a pedometer as motivational tools to promote more activity through increasing the number of steps taken daily. It is based on awareness, motivational approaches, and elimination of barriers to move people through stages of achievement from low activity (about 4,000 steps) to a higher daily level of activity (about 10,000 steps). **Contact:** HealthPartners, **www.healthpartners.com**.

REFERENCES AND RESOURCES

1. Foo, MA, Robinson, J, Rhodes, M, Lew, LS, Chao, M, Dy, SS, Eir, W. Identifying policy opportunities to increase physical activity in the Southeast Asian community in Long Beach, California. *Journal of Health Education*, 1999; 30(2 Supplement): S58-S63.

2. Lindberg, Rebecca, MPH, RD. Active living: On the road with the 10,000 Steps program. *Journal of The American Dietetic Association*, 2000; 100(8).

3. Fletcher GF, Balady G, Blair SN, Blumenthal J, Caspersen C, Chaitman B, Epstein S, Froelicher ESS, Froelicher VF, Pina IL, Pollock ML. Statement on Exercise: Benefits and Recommendations for Physical Activity Programs for All Americans. American Heart Association Medical/Scientific Statement, 1996.

4. Glanz, K, Mullis, RM. Environmental interventions to promote healthy eating: a review of models, programs and evidence. *Health Education Quarterly*, 1988; 15(4): 395-415.

5. Bogden, JF, Vega-Matos, CA. Fit, healthy, and ready to learn: A school health policy guide. Part 1: Physical activity, healthy eating, and tobacco-use prevention. 2000.

6. Frank, LD, Engelke, P. How Land Use and Transportation Systems Impact Public Health: A Literature Review of the Relationship between Physical Activity and Built Form. ACE's Working Paper #1. CDC, 2000: 147 pp.

7. *Physical Activity and Health: A Report of the Surgeon General*. CDC, 1996. Superintendent of Documents. S/N 017-023-00196-5.

8. Sallis, JF, et al. The association of school environments with youth physical activity. *American Journal of Public Health*, April 2001; 91(4): 618-620.

9. Cohen, J. Overweight Kids: Why Should We Care? California Research Bureau, 2000: 1-42.

10. IOM, Promoting Health Intervention Strategies for Social and Behavioral Research. National Academy Press, Washington, DC, 2000.

11. Siegel, M, Doner, L. Marketing public health: strategies to promote social change. Aspen Publications, Gaithersburg, MD, 1998.

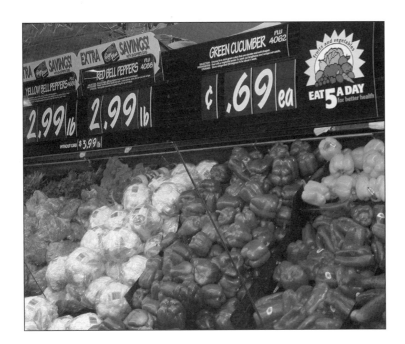

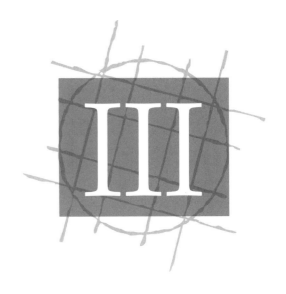

Mass Communication

The mass media, media advocacy, and public relations allow us not only to get healthy eating and physical activity messages out to large groups of people but also to frame issues and focus on policy and systems change. Through the media, people become aware of the resources available to help them and are shown how making healthy changes can improve their lives. When we research media messages properly and present them effectively, those messages can alter the community's attitudes toward healthy practices, which ultimately can lead to changes in public policy as well.

RATIONALE

For major shifts in a population's behavior and norms, utilizing the process and the tools of marketing and mass communication are essential. Mass media interventions can reach almost every member of a society. They can help to unify social action and drive consumer demand for healthy eating, physical activity services, and changes in the environment and public policy. Media interventions support community programs, raise visibility, and help sustain behavior change. Media and marketing are essential tools in the overall comprehensive approach. Communication plans must be based on consumer research for the segments of interest, using surveys, focus groups, and other qualitative research directed at the intended audiences.

SAMPLE ACTIVITIES

1. Qualitative and quantitative research identifies information about the problem to be addressed, the target audience, knowledge, attitudes, behavior, relevant social issues, and the larger context.

2. Mass media campaigns emphasize healthful eating and physical activity patterns, a shift in social norms, and a systems/policy change.

3. Paid, cooperative, and public service advertising (e.g., broadcast, print, outdoor, transit) increases public awareness in the general market and the targeted market segments that include ethnic- and income-specific groups, and children and youth.

4. Public relations activities support partner activities, generate free media coverage, and secure premium placement of public service advertising.

5. Seasonal or theme promotions generate fresh interest and organize action for institutional or consumer behavior change.

6. Media advocacy and civic journalism drive policy change.

7. Social science, communication, and marketing theory guide message development, audience, and channel selection.

8. Deliver pretested strategies and messages to members of the audience.

9. Evaluate message dissemination for reach, frequency, and duration with the target audience as compared against goals for target rating points.

10. Use multimedia, including the Internet, toll-free numbers, small media, brochures, posters, and fillers.

11. Use awards and recognition for socially responsible advertising practices by media outlets, food and physical activity companies, and other partners.

Sample Practices and Programs

1% or Less Campaign—Multiple messages and activities are used to influence communities to increase consumption of low-fat milk. A feature of the campaign is the *1% or Less School Kit*, which contains materials for primary and secondary school students: idea sheets, fact sheets, marketing strategies, model press releases, handouts, posters, and instructions for conducting taste tests. **Contact:** Center for Science in the Public Interest, **www.cspinet.org/kids**, 202-332-9110.

5-a-Day for Better Health—These campaigns, implemented in most states, increase public awareness of the importance of eating more fruits and vegetables for better health. Offered through a collaboration between NIH and the Produce for Better Health Foundation, components include a retailer point-of-purchase educational program, a food service educational program, and a national media program. The national 5-a-Day program will undergo significant expansion in 2002. **Contact:** National Cancer Institute, **www.5aday.gov**, Produce for Better Health Foundation, **www.5aday.com**, 302-738-7100.

Eat Smart, Play Hard—This campaign is designed to foster positive changes in eating and physical activity behaviors targeting children ages 2 to 18 and their caregivers. The campaign themes focus on breakfast, snacks, balance, and physical activity. Suggested activities are consistent with the Dietary Guidelines for Americans and the Food Guide Pyramid. **Contact:** USDA Food and Nutrition Service, **www.fns.usda.gov/FNS/mascot/mascot.htm**.

REFERENCES AND RESOURCES

1. Making Health Communication Programs Work: A Planner's Guide. NIH Publication 89-1493:131.
2. Caroll, A, Craypo, L, Samuels, S. Evaluating Nutrition and Physical Activity Social Marketing Campaigns: A Review of the Literature for Use in Community Campaigns. Center for Advanced Studies in Nutrition and Social Marketing, University of California at Davis, 2000.
3. Sims, LS, Randell, JS, Haas, E. Comprehensive Review of the Effectiveness of Nutrition Education Interventions with Target Audiences. *The Journal of Nutrition Education,* 1995; 27(6).
4. Building Media Skills for Better Nutrition. Videoconference Guide, CDC, 1994: 1-35.
5. Contento, I, et al. Theoretical Frameworks or Models for Nutrition Education. *The Journal of Nutrition Education,* 1995; 27 (6).

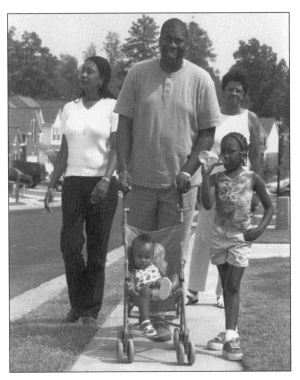

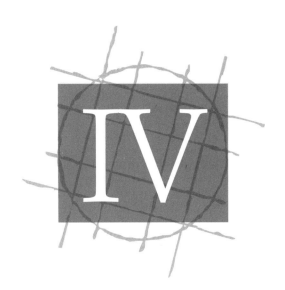

Community Programs and Community Development

Communities can promote healthy eating and physical activity among their residents by creating the necessary infrastructure and economic development for those behaviors. However, those in the community must participate with nonprofit, philanthropic, and business sectors to make this happen. Whether interventions take the form of building more recreational areas, providing safe places for exercise, or making public policy that favors healthier food choices, planned development that comes from individuals in the community can assist people in living healthier lifestyles.

RATIONALE

Building an infrastructure to support healthy diets and regular physical activity requires a commitment to developing and sustaining health promoting policies, resources, and practices. Healthy communities are in a dynamic state of renewal, continually creating and improving their physical and social environments and enabling all of their citizens to make healthy choices. An engaged citizenry is the core element of a strong community infrastructure.

The social, political, and cultural environments in communities affect the knowledge, beliefs, attitudes, and behaviors related to diet and physical activity of all members. Effective community programs involve people in their homes, worksites, schools, places of worship and entertainment, civic organizations, and other public places. Community-based interventions involve the community in planning and creating environments that make the healthy choice the easiest choice for eating and physical activity. Community programs should focus on four goals:

1. Provide opportunities to learn how to be active, how to eat healthfully, and how to

maintain a healthy weight among people of all ages.

2. Provide safe environments for physical activity.

3. Provide accessible and affordable opportunities for all people to be active and eat healthfully.

4. Eliminate disparities in support and resources for physical activity and healthy eating.

These goals can be achieved by community programs that

- increase the number of citizens and organizations who are involved in planning and conducting community programs and who participate in other related community activities, such as transportation, park, and land use planning;

- organize disenfranchised groups and advocate equity in health (e.g., strengthening food security programs or organizing community groups to demand secure recreation areas);

- use state and local social marketing, media advocacy, and countermarketing campaigns that inform, educate, and engage citizens about nutrition, physical activity, and obesity-related policies and issues in their communities;

- promote the adoption of public and private food and physical activity policies and community infrastructure (e.g., sidewalks, farmers markets, retail grocers, and public health impact statements to support healthy eating and physical activity); and

- measure outcomes using a range of surveillance and evaluation techniques.

SAMPLE ACTIVITIES

1. Promote sustained physical activity lifestyles for adults and children, such as brisk walking or cycling, as defined by national guidelines (e.g., CDC/ACSM guidelines). (See Pate et al. 1995.)

2. Use multiple channels for interventions, such as retail food outlets, transit and recreation/leisure facilities, worksites, and social service centers to reach the general population and targeted subgroups within the community.

3. Coordinate community-wide, geographically specific, or multichannel projects—like coalitions, planning, and lateral integration—that use community development and consumer empowerment approaches. This strategy includes initial assessments with environmental scans, goal setting, and feedback loop.

4. Create advocacy and policy projects that fully utilize available federal food assistance programs for children, seniors, and low-income persons and state-specific resources, such as increasing participation in the food stamp program and increasing the availability and quality of the school breakfast and lunch programs.

5. Conduct community-wide healthy eating and physical activity special events, regular programming, and media campaigns.

6. Change zoning and land use requirements to mandate sidewalks, trails, safe pedestrian and bicycle access to schools, shopping, parks, and recreation centers.

7. Allow vending machines and cafeterias on school property to offer only healthy foods and drinks.

8. Keep schools and grounds open before and after school hours for public use, and offer after-school activity programs that are accessible and affordable for all students.

9. Promote governmental and nongovernmental organization policies that promote physical activity and healthy eating (e.g., at worksites, places of worship, at meetings, in health insurance coverage).

10. Promote increased bicycling by providing bike parking in front of buildings and in public spaces and by also providing bike carriers and access on buses, light rail, and other public transportation.

Sample Practices and Programs

Missouri Department of Health Community Physical Activity Programs—Working with the Missouri Department of Health and the Saint Louis University Prevention Research Center, community coalitions in southeast Missouri conducted a needs assessment, then planned and constructed 13 community walking trails, and concluded the project by conducting follow-up interviews and surveys of trail users and community residents. The trails stimulated increased activity and access to safe activity for residents. **Contact:** Ross Brownson, **brownson@slu.edu**, 314-977-8110.

Cool Kids—This project in Virginia educates parents of overweight two- to four-year-old children enrolled in the WIC program about the benefits of healthier eating and improved physical activity for their children. Parents learn to purchase more nutritious foods, to encourage healthier snacking habits, and to influence their children to be more engaged in play instead of watching television. **Contact:** Virginia Department of Health, **kheise@vdh. state.va.us**.

Zuni Wellness Center—A comprehensive program emphasizing healthful lifestyles for the prevention of diabetes, hypertension, dyslipidemia, and alcoholism. The most successful and established component is the Zuni Fitness Series, emphasizing nutrition and physical activity. **Contact:** Zuni Wellness Center, **gloria.lucero@mail.ihs.gov**.

Michigan Fitness Foundation—The goal of this program is to finance and support physical fitness, health, and sports through public information, fundraising, curriculum development, coalitions, and partnerships. A statewide network of Regional Councils on Physical Fitness, Health, and Sports has been implemented and several projects are under way. **Contact:** Michigan Fitness Foundation, **www.michiganfitness. org**.

Arthritis Self-Help Course—Developed at Stanford University, this course has been demonstrated effectively with Hispanic populations in Florida. The Florida Department of Health's Arthritis Prevention and Education Program worked with community-based organizations to teach the course in group settings while encouraging increased physical activity. Results have shown a reduction of arthritis pain by 20% and a reduction of physician visits by 40%. **Contact:** Heather Murphy, **heather_ murphy@doh.state.fl.us**.

Healthy Indian Kids Exercise Study (HIKES)— Designed to reduce obesity and diabetes in children, this program in southwest Oklahoma engages community residents, physical education teachers, and parents to teach children about healthy food choices, to negotiate the use of school athletic facilities for after-school

hours, and to supervise after-school free play and team sports.

Contact: William Moore, **william-moore @ouhsc.edu**, 405-271-2330.

Protective Life Corporation Workplace Wellness Program—This worksite program in Alabama provides an environment to enhance employee skills to achieve wellness and to create a culture that encourages healthy lifestyles. An employee "pro-health team" provides ideas and energy for the program. Health assessments, health education, fitness and sports activities, nutrition consultation, "free fruit" days, health screening, and physical activity incentives are provided. **Contact:** Protective Life Corporation, 800-866-3555, ext. 3129.

Sisters Together: Move More, Eat Better— The goals of this program are to encourage personal change, support normative changes, and strengthen and expand local resources to prevent obesity. An information campaign is wrapped within a community development model with an emphasis on social marketing. Activities include tip sheets, recipes, stories, a walking booklet, hair care tips for exercising women, and a resource guide. A manual is also available. **Contact:** Sisters Together, **www.hsph. harvard.edu/sisterstogether**.

California Adolescent Nutrition and Fitness (CANFit)—A comprehensive program to improve the nutritional status and physical fitness of low-income African American, American Indian, Latino, and Asian/Pacific Islander youths, ages 10 to 14. Local projects build community leadership; implement multilevel interventions; leverage additional resources; provide scholarships to study nutrition, physical activity, public health, or culinary arts; and evaluate and disseminate viable projects. Program materials include proposal guidelines, bibliographies, a guidebook, and a newsletter. **Contact:** California Adolescent Nutrition and Fitness Program, **www.canfit.org**, 510-644-1533.

REFERENCES AND RESOURCES

1. Truman, BI, Smith-Akin, CK, Hinman, AR, et al., and the Task Force on Community Preventive Services. Developing the Guide to Community Preventive Services' Overview and Rationale. *American Journal of Preventive Medicine*, 2000; 18(supplement 1).

2. Fawcett, SB, Francisco, VT, Schultz, JA, Berkowitz, B, Wolff, TJ, Nagy, G. Community Tool Box: A Web-Based Resource for Building Healthier Communities. *Public Health Reports*, March-April and May-June, 2000; 115: 274-278.

3. Donahue, RP, Abbott, RD, Reed, DM, Yano, K. Physical Activity and Coronary Heart Disease in Middle-Aged and Elderly Men: The Honolulu Heart Program. *American Journal of Public Health*, 1988; 78(6): 683-685.

4. Improving America's Diet and Health-From Recommendations to Action. A Report of the Committee on Dietary Guidelines Implementation. IOM, 1991.

5. The ProHealth Wellness Program (brochure). Protective Life Corporation, Birmingham, AL, 2001.

6. Promoting Physical Activity: A Guide for Community Action. CDC. Champaign, IL: Human Kinetics, 1999.

7. The National Bicycling and Walking Study: Transportation Choices for a Changing America. Final Report. Federal Highway Administration, US DOT, 1994.

8. On the Move—California's Physical Activity Initiative, *Journal of Health Education*, March/April 1999; 30(2): 1-71(S).

9. Probert, K.L. (Ed.). Moving to the Future: Developing Community-Based Nutrition Services. Washington, DC: Association of State and Territorial Public Health Nutrition Directors, 1996.

10. How to Promote Physical Activity in Your Community, 1996. 2nd ed. Physical Activity Workgroup (PAWG), December 1997.

11. Pate, et al. Physical activity and public health. A recommendation for the Centers for Disease Control and Prevention and the American College of Sports Medicine. *Journal of the American Medical Association*, 1995 Feb 1; 273(5): 402-407.

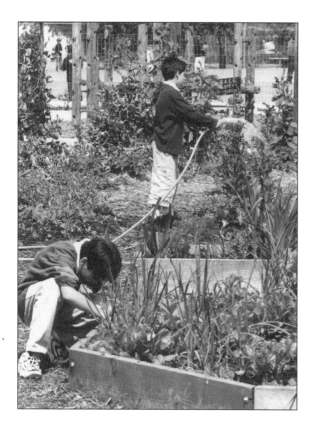

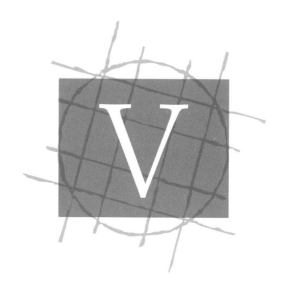

Programs for Children and Youth

While young people are more at risk than ever before for obesity, diabetes, and the accompanying health problems, the opportunities for them to make healthy choices have also diminished. Many of the school and community programs that used to support children's health, such as daily physical education, are often no longer available. What adds to the problem is the lure of sedentary pursuits, such as television and video games, and the availability of high-calorie, low-nutrition foods in competition with nutritious school lunches. Through community, school, and business-based partners, we need to offer programs for this age group that will keep them interested in physical activity and promote good nutrition.

RATIONALE

Young people build healthy bodies and establish healthy lifestyles by being physically active and eating healthily in their daily lives. However, few young people meet recommendations for good health; a minority is physically active on a regular basis; and both physical activity and dietary quality decline in adolescence.

Two periods of life have been identified as strategic in the development of childhood obesity. First, during the prenatal period, excess maternal weight gain, gestational diabetes, and high birth weight are factors that raise the risk of obesity later in life. Second, being at risk or overweight in adolescence has a very high risk of persisting into adulthood.

Recommended family strategies include increasing the duration of breastfeeding, controlling television time, and restoring balance to the parent-child feeding relationship. Maternal, child, and adolescent programs such as Head Start, WIC, and school-based programs have the opportunity to target more intensive dietary guidance and physical activity guidance to parents, caretakers, and young people.

At the same time that obesity rates rise, the number of students enrolled in daily school-based and school-linked programs to develop lifelong physical activity patterns is decreasing. From 1991 to 1995, participation in daily physical education programs in high schools dropped from 42% to 25%. School reform initiatives that focus exclusively on academics have squeezed time from school days formerly reserved for physical education programs. Computers, video games, cable television, and other more sedentary pursuits compete for the leisure time of young people. Food environments have an abundance of foods high in fat and sugar with limited healthier food options. Many schools offer competitive or à la carte foods as alternatives to nutritious school lunches, thereby encouraging unhealthy eating habits. Competitive foods such as soft drinks, chips, candy, and fast-food courts in schools that contribute to the lack of healthy choices for students are driven in many school districts by the need for revenues realized through these high-margin offerings.

Recommended intervention sites include the following:

• Within families and in community settings, opportunities for physical activity can be increased through walking, bicycling, and other forms of recreation and free play. This intervention may include providing more recreational equipment and adult supervision for after-school, weekend, and summer competitive and recreational activity or improving walking and biking routes between residential areas and schools.

• Schools (preschools, child care, K-12) should offer daily physical activity of sufficient duration and intensity for all children, provide healthier foods, and reduce or eliminate competitive foods of minimum or low-nutrient value that are sold on campus. If competitive foods are offered, then they should represent choices from the five major food groups of the food guide.

• In medical settings, pediatricians and other providers can promote healthy nutrition and physical activity habits.

• Worksites can help parents to be more active and, in turn, encourage more physical activity among family members.

• Community-wide mass media targeted to children and adolescents can deliver important messages about healthful eating and regular physical activity.

SAMPLE ACTIVITIES

1. Provide regular opportunities for all children and youth to engage in physical activity and healthy eating behaviors, as well as to develop the knowledge, skills, and attitudes necessary for lifelong engagement in these behaviors.

2. Work with preschool and child care partners to strengthen policies that ensure adequate physical activity and healthy food choices.

3. Help underwrite school-centered programs and campaigns at four developmental levels: lower elementary, upper elementary, middle school, and high school.

4. Encourage community initiatives with youth organizations, businesses, and programs after school and during the summer.

5. Collaborate with media and advertising industries to promote more positive advertising to children and youth.

6. Promote a continuum of physical activity from early childhood through adolescence that is sequential and developmentally appropriate.

7. Improve promotion of healthy eating and physical activity in primary care settings, including adoption of anticipatory prevention guidance and breast-feeding promotion strategies and guidelines.

8. Create intermediary linkages, including teacher and staff incentives and training.

9. Set school policy and standards that reflect national health objectives for nutrition and physical activity.

Sample Practices and Programs

CATCH (Coordinated Approach to School Health)—a multilevel, multicomponent intervention to promote a healthy school environment as well as improve healthy eating behaviors and physical activity levels for students in grades K-5. Positive changes in knowledge, attitudes, and behaviors have been reported from trials and have been sustained during the three-year period of involvement in the program. Lesson plans, workbooks, and videos are available. **Contact:** Guy Parcell, 713-792-8547.

SPARK—This is a physical education curriculum and staff development program for students in grades K-6. Students from third grade to sixth grade are engaged in a self-management curriculum that includes in-school and family participation. A SPARK staff member trains teachers through workshops and follow-up consultations. Improvements in levels of physical performance were observed for SPARK students compared with controls for a period of two years after intervention. Materials include a set of physical education and self-management textbooks. **Contact:** 800-SPARK PE, **www.foundation.sdsu.edu/projects/spark/index.html**.

Planet Health—The Harvard Prevention Research Center created this curriculum that integrates health messages into physical activity sessions and lessons in social studies, science, language arts, and math. The curriculum has been piloted in Boston public schools. **Contact:** Jean Wiecha,

jwiecha@hsph.harvard.edu, 617-432-4255.

San Luis Valley Community Coalition—This Colorado project brings schools, community resources, and three generations of family members together to build a school environment that supports healthful eating and physical activity. Components of the program are parent volunteers for lunchtime sessions on healthy eating, training Boys and Girls Club mentors for diet and activity, and training lay health facilitators to visit with families. **Contact:** Julie Marshall, **julie.marshall@uhsc.edu**, 303-315-7596.

A World Fit for Kids—This program was developed in a violent Los Angeles neighborhood. It engages youth to become mentor coaches, and with the help of program coordinators, they then engage elementary through high school youth in fitness activities to build self-esteem, teach conflict resolution, and foster leadership skills. The program champion and role model is Kevin Sorbo, star of the *Hercules* television show. He stimulates the formation of coalitions to gain volunteers for the program. **Contact:** A World Fit for Kids, **www.worldfitforkids.org/aafsorbo.html**, 213-387-7712.

Project Fit America—This program aims to increase awareness of the benefits of regular physical activity at the elementary school level and to enhance overall health and well-being. The project provides comprehensive fitness equipment, educational in-services for teachers, and a curriculum guide for classroom lessons. Local businesses are engaged to provide the equipment for the project, and volunteers are recruited to supplement the staff. Children participating in the project show marked increases in fitness. **Contact:** Project Fit America, **www.projectfitamerica.org**.

Changing the Scene: Improving the School Nutrition Environment, A Guide to Local Action—This is toolkit developed by USDA's Food and Nutrition Service to help communities promote healthy school nutrition. It features a guide that offers practical advice on taking local action to improve school nutrition as well as background materials explaining the importance of healthy eating to children's long-term health and well-being. The kit also includes handouts, sample materials, a video, and a PowerPoint presentation. **Contact:** **www.fns.usda.gov**.

REFERENCES AND RESOURCES

1. Youth Risk Behavior Surveillance—United States, 1999. Morbidity and Mortality Weekly Report, U.S. Centers for Disease Control and Prevention, June 9, 2000.
2. Physical Activity and Good Nutrition: Essential Elements for Good Health. At-a-Glance Document. U.S. Centers for Disease Control and Prevention, 1999.
3. Unrealized Prevention Opportunities: Reducing the Health and Economic Burden of Chronic Disease. National Center for Chronic Disease Prevention and Health Promotion, U.S. Centers for Disease Control and Prevention, March 1997.
4. Moving into the Future: National Standards for Physical Education. National Association for Sport and Physical Education, 1995.
5. Walk Our Children to School Day. Partnership for a Walkable America, National Safety Council, Department of Transportation. **www.walktoschool-usa.org/**
6. Guidelines for School Health Programs to Promote Lifelong Healthy Eating. CDC. MMWR, 1996; 45(RR-9): 1-41.
7. Guidelines for School and Community Programs to Promote Lifelong Physical Activity Among Young People. CDC. MMWR, 1997; 46(RR-6).

8. Promoting Better Health for Young People Through Physical Activity and Sports: A Report to the President from the Secretary of Health and Human Services and the Secretary of Education. CDC, 2000.

9. Kids-Walk-to-School: A Guide for Community Action to Promote Children Walking to School. CDC, 2000.

10. USDA, Food and Nutrition Service, Office of Analysis, Nutrition and Evaluation, School Nutrition Dietary Assessment Study-II Final Report. CH-01-SNDAIIFR, by Mary Kay Fox, et al. Project Officer, Patricia McKinney. Alexandria, VA: 2001. **www.fns.usda.gov/MENU/Published/CNP/FILES/SMIYear1.pdf**

11. USDA, Food and Nutrition Service, Office of Analysis, Nutrition and Evaluation, School Meals Initiative Implementation Study-First Year Report, SN-00-SMI1, by Sameer Abraham et al. Project Director, John Endahl, Patricia McKinney. Alexandria, VA: 2000. **www.fns.usda.gov/oane/MENU/Published/CNP/FILES/smiy2.pdf**

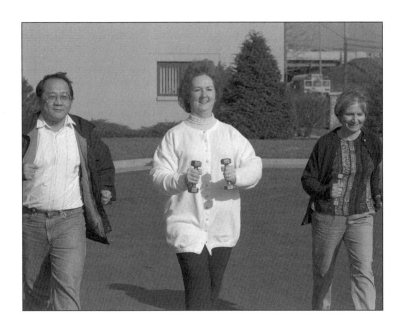

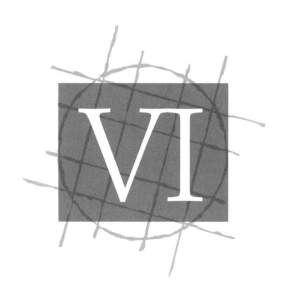

Health Care Delivery

Many people look to their physicians and other health care workers for guidance on health matters; thus, the involvement of health care delivery systems in promoting healthy lifestyles is a natural link. The focus of that involvement should be preventive measures, which may include advice on eating and physical activity, testing for disease risk factors, referrals for treatment, and partnering with other community organizations for health promotion.

RATIONALE

Health care delivery systems can play an important role in promoting physical activity and healthy eating as well as treating overweight and obesity through a variety of methods such as counseling, referral, research, and the provision of incentives and benefits.

Prevention must be emphasized as the most effective and cost-effective approach to avoid-

ing the mortality and morbidity associated with obesity and a sedentary lifestyle. Interventions need to be implemented that encourage children, adolescents, and adults to develop life-long habits that lead to a healthy eating style, active living, and healthy weight. This movement will take the cooperation and commitment of parents, schools, communities, health care providers, and managed care or other health care funding sources to promote positive change in personal health behavior, social norms, and the food and activity environments. Change must be socially acceptable, economically sustainable, and culturally appropriate.

In addition to prevention activities, strategies are needed to provide the assistance and funding for the weight loss and weight management of obese children and adults to control chronic diseases and reduce medication costs. Even modest weight loss in obese adults—between 5% and 10% of body weight—have been shown to improve glucose tolerance, hyperlipidemia, and blood pressure. Regular physical activity substantially reduces the risk of dying of coronary heart disease; it decreases the risk for colon cancer, diabetes, and high blood pressure; it helps to control weight; it contributes to healthy bones, muscles, and joints; and it reduces symptoms of anxiety and depression.

Programs that successfully motivate or assist people to eat healthier and be more physically active are the cornerstones in the prevention and control of obesity in both children and adults. To reverse the current public heath epidemic of obesity, the health care delivery system must implement policies and cost-effective programs to improve the health and the quality of life for every citizen.

The Medicare program has recently added medical nutrition therapy as a benefit, and some managed care plans include policies and procedures to promote nutrition and physical activity education and treatment services. Primary and secondary components in health care settings should include the following objectives:

- Establish priorities for anticipatory guidance in primary care to promote among healthy people, such as eating five fruits and vegetables per day, drinking 1% (or less) fat milk, or getting 30 to 60 minutes of physical activity each day.
- Establish priorities for secondary prevention—for example, the early detection and reversal of risk factors such as elevated blood lipids, high blood pressure, high blood sugar, and weight gain—and include referral to community resources.
- Assess patients and subscribers for their interests in nutrition and physical activity education and self-care; conduct record audits; and determine opportunities for services with potential cost savings.
- Assess the community for assets and needs, such as access to healthy food and to physical activity facilities, and to organizations to partner with for public awareness campaigns, special events, and environmental change.
- In fee-for-service health systems, establish referral and billing procedures for physical therapy and medical nutrition therapy.

SAMPLE ACTIVITIES

1. Establish and promote standards of practice, quality assurance for managed care, and other health care delivery systems such as the *Guide to Clinical Preventive Services*.

2. Provide and promote reimbursement for services of registered dietitians or other proven interventions for nutrition, physical activity, and obesity treatment as per the Institute of Medicine Report recommendations for heart attack, stroke, and diabetes.

3. Establish collaboration with public and private health plans to establish a common set of preventive benefits that reduce the risk pool of the total population.

4. Adopt the clinical preventive guidance from the resources *Bright Futures in Practice: Nutrition* and *Bright Futures in Practice: Physical Activity*.

5. Utilize the Baby Friendly Hospital Initiative to improve breastfeeding initiation and duration rates.

Sample Practices and Programs

KidShape—A family-centered pediatric weight management program, developed in response to the development of type 2 diabetes in Los Angeles youth. This program involves the family in basic education and counseling coupled with physician-directed activities to guide obese youth. Some elements of the program are being reimbursed through MediCal. **Contact:** Naomi Neufeld, **ndneufeld@pol.net**.

A New Leaf—This program, developed at the University of North Carolina, is a structured nutrition, physical activity, and smoking cessation assessment and intervention program for cardiovascular disease reduction among low-income individuals. New Leaf integrates behavior change theory with nutrition and exercise science in a clinically feasible intervention tool. **Contact:** New Leaf Intervention, **www.hpdp.unc.edu/wisewoman**.

Bright Futures—These guidelines for professionals provide practical information, effective preventive techniques, and health promotion materials for health supervision of infants, children, and adolescents. The materials include a nutrition guide, a physical activity guide, and information about iron deficiency anemia screening, hyperlipidemia screening, and hypertension screening. **Contact:** National Maternal and Child Health Clearinghouse, **www.brightfutures.org**.

Baby Friendly Hospital Initiative—This program recognizes hospitals and birth centers that have taken steps to provide an optimal environment for the promotion, protection, and support of breast-feeding. Hospitals receive the "Baby-Friendly" designation when they successfully implement the WHO/UNICEF "Ten Steps to Successful Breastfeeding." **Contact:** Baby-Friendly USA, **www.babyfriendlyusa.org**.

Committed to Kids Pediatric Weight Management Program—an integrated, multidisciplinary team approach to preventing and treating obesity in children. Four program components are conducted in group sessions with support from family and others. Training and consultation staff members are available. Curriculum guides and a procedures manual are available. Contact: **www.committed-to-kids.com**.

REFERENCES AND RESOURCES

1. Barlow, SE, Dietz, WH. Obesity evaluation and treatment: Expert committee recommendations. *Pediatrics*, 1998; 102(3).

2. Recommendation to Prevent and Control Iron Deficiency in the United States. CDC. MMWR, 1998; 47(RR-3): 1-29.

3. HHS Blueprint for Action on Breastfeeding. DHHS Office on Women's Health, 2000.

4. Preventing Obesity Among Children. Chronic Disease Notes and Reports, CDC, 2000; 13(1).

5. U.S. Preventive Services Task Force. Guide to Clinical Preventive Services, 2d ed. Alexandria, VA: International Medical Publishing, 1996.

6. National Heart, Lung, and Blood Institute Expert Panel on the Identification, Evaluation, and Treatment of Overweight and Obesity in Adults, *Executive summary of the clinical guidelines on the identification, evaluation, and treatment of overweight and obesity in adults. JADA*, October 1998; 98(10): 1178-1191.

7. Rippe, JM, Hess, S. The Role of Physical Activity in the Prevention and Management of Obesity. *JADA*, 1998; 98(suppl 2): S31-S38.

8. Thompson, D, Edelsberg, J, Kinsey, KL, and Oster, G. Estimated Economic Costs of Obesity to US Business. *American Journal of Health Promotion*, November/December 1998; 13: 120-127.

9. Troiano, RP, Flegal, KM, Kuczmarski, RJ, Campbell, SM, Johnson, CL. *Overweight Prevalence and Trends for Children and Adolescents, The National Health and Nutrition Examination Surveys, 1963 to 1991*. Arch. Pediatr. Adolesc. Med. 1995; 149: 1085-1091.

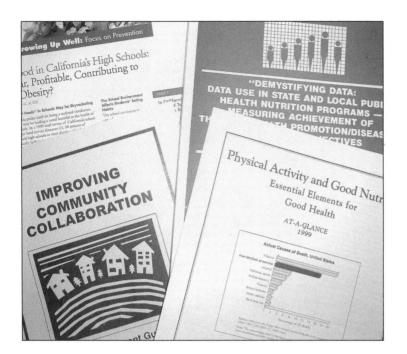

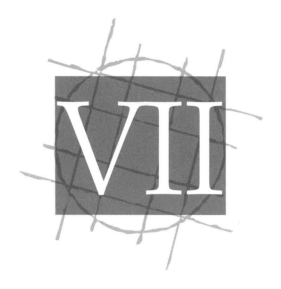

Surveillance, Epidemiology, and Research

Accurate data are needed to guide the formation of programs that will improve the public's health behaviors and to assess the success of those programs. We require several different methods to identify state and community needs and attitudes, to determine priorities and actions, to test interventions, and to evaluate progress. We should include state-level surveys and formative research in ongoing data collection.

RATIONALE

Surveillance and epidemiology are essential public health tools for monitoring trends, setting priorities, conducting statewide planning, mobilizing action, allocating resources, forming policy decisions for local grants, and evaluating results. Systems of surveillance and research that focus on the trends, antecedents, and deter-

minants (particularly behavioral and environmental determinants) of eating, exercise, and obesity are needed for tracking the incidence of overweight and obesity and for measuring and evaluating the impact of efforts to modify behavioral risk factors. A mix of survey, surveillance, and qualitative research systems—including social marketing research—is needed. Data sources to design, implement, and evaluate a comprehensive nutrition, physical activity, and obesity control need to be identified.

SAMPLE ACTIVITIES

1. Develop the scientific capacity to assess in the priority population(s) the burden of poor nutrition, inactivity, obesity, and related chronic diseases. Data systems should monitor trends, disseminate data and information, and support evaluation efforts.

2. Develop or identify surveillance and evaluation strategies to monitor environmental and policy measures relevant to the plan's objectives, such as auditing the physical activity resources in a community or the low-fat foods available in stores.

3. Measure availability and utilization of parks, open space, green space, pocket parks, and alternative transportation.

4. Identify and assess existing and desired sources of data for use in the development and enhancement of surveillance system(s) to monitor (at minimum) body mass index (BMI), dietary, and physical activity behaviors in the priority population(s).

5. Undertake alternative surveillance strategies to address state or community-specific unmet surveillance needs—for example, oversampling, special surveys, sentinel surveillance systems, "stand-alone" telephone surveys, or other state-specific surveys and surveillance systems such as representative surveys of children and public opinion polling.

6. Develop and implement a review process for considering changes in current surveillance systems to address state, regional, and local data needs.

7. Allocate resources and staff time toward surveillance, data management, evaluation, and other activities associated with surveillance and evaluation efforts.

8. Conduct studies to examine situational and environmental variables for all age groups.

9. Undertake qualitative research or use existing research to understand consumer segments and intermediaries. Techniques include focus groups, key informant interviews, ethnographic mapping, media tracking and content analysis, opinion leader reviews, theater testing, and mall intercept studies.

10. Conduct consumer research to identify audiences, pilot test new initiatives, evaluate interventions, and transfer new technologies to different settings or population segments. This objective may be met by the state program or through contract with an academic center, market research company, or university.

Sample Practices and Programs

California High School Fast Food Survey— This survey documented types of fast food sold on California high school campuses, the factors that influence such sales, and the economic and policy issues associated with them. The survey was conducted in 171 school districts representing 345 high schools. The survey concluded that over the past 10 years, fast foods have become a staple on high school campuses. **Contact:** The Public Health Institute, **www.phi.org**, Select newsroom 510-644-8200.

1999 California Children's Eating and Exercise Practices Survey—This survey was conducted in April and June 1999 by the California Endowment and the U.S. Department of Agriculture. A sample of parents assisted their 9- to 11-year-old children to maintain a two-day food and physical activity diary. A total of 814 children completed the survey. Results showed that children who participated in school lunch and breakfast programs ate more fruit and vegetable servings, and children who were overweight or at risk for overweight ate fewer fruit and vegetable servings than normal-weight children. Physically inactive children also consumed fewer servings than active children consumed. **Contact:** The Public Health Institute, **www.phi.org**, Select newsroom 510-644-8200.

Wateree Health District Physical Activity Assessments—The Santee Healthy People Coalition worked with the South Carolina Department of Health and Environmental Control and the Prevention Research Center to assess the environment for promotion of physical activity. This research included community interviews about assets, needs and values, inventory of existing physical activity programs offered in the community, and conduct of windshield tours and walkability audits to assess community resources and supports. This information is being used to train community teams and to develop collaborative strategies to improve physical activity. **Contact:** Barbara Ainsworth, **http://prevention.sph.sc.edu**, 803-777-4253.

REFERENCES AND RESOURCES

1. Centers for Disease Control and Prevention. Framework for Program Evaluation in Public Health. MMWR, 1999; 48(No. RR-11).
2. Centers for Disease Control and Prevention. School Health Index for Physical Activity and Healthy Eating: A Self-Assessment and Planning Guide: Middle School/High School. 2000. **www.cdc.gov**
3. Centers for Disease Control and Prevention. School Health Index for Physical Activity and Healthy Eating: A Self-Assessment and Planning Guide: Elementary School. 2000. **www.cdc.gov**
4. Healthy Weight, Physical Activity, and Nutrition: Focus Group Research with African American, Mexican American, and White Youth. Executive Summary, CDC, June 2000.

APPENDIX A

Funding Case Studies for Nutrition and Physical Activity Programs

The following two case studies describe funding, strategies, and activities from two states at significantly different developmental stages with respect to their programs for nutrition and physical activity. The Hawaii case study describes how that state, through the Healthy Hawaii Initiative, plans to utilize a recent major allocation from the tobacco settlement funds. The California case study describes, in the context of the seven components discussed in this document, how nutrition and physical activity programs in that state have been supported through the California Nutrition Network since fiscal year (FY) 1996-97.

HAWAII CASE STUDY

The 20th state legislature of Hawaii established the Hawaii Tobacco Settlement Special Fund within the state treasury, administered by the Department of Health (DOH). This legislation mandates that 25% of the monies in the Tobacco Settlement Special Fund be used for health promotion and disease prevention programs. To fulfill this mandate, and in keeping with its mission, the Department of Health of the state of Hawaii has established the Healthy Hawaii Initiative (HHI) to provide leadership to monitor, promote, protect, and enhance the health and environmental well-being of all of Hawaii's people. This initiative is a major statewide effort to encourage healthy lifestyles and the environments to support them.

The intent of the HHI is to use the tobacco settlement funds to provide the over 1.2 million residents of Hawaii with the information and technical assistance needed to promote improved health. The major goals of the initiative are to (1) increase quality and years of healthy life for Hawaii's people and (2) reduce existing health disparities among ethnic groups in Hawaii. HHI includes three primary focus areas—tobacco prevention and control, physical activity promotion, and nutrition. The HHI represents the Hawaii DOH's long-term strategic planning for environmental and policy-related efforts in these areas. It does not provide personal health care services.

The HHI has four major components that will seek to accomplish the following goals:

1. School-based initiatives

2. Healthy communities initiatives

3. Public and professional education

4. Hawaii Outcomes Institute for Assessment and Evaluation

A significant proportion of the funding for these components is provided from the tobacco settlement funds. The current budget is allocated through FY 2003. The FY 2001 allocation ceiling is $9.6 million; the FY 2002 ceiling is $9.5 million; and the FY 2003 ceiling is $12.46 million. Additionally, the tobacco settlement funds provide approximately $300,000 annually for enforcement activities related to tobacco. Although the tobacco master settlement speaks to 25 years of funding to settling states, the Hawaii Department of Health is preparing for a possible shorter funding cycle of approximately 10 years. The department will use current tobacco settlement funding as seed money to prepare the model to leverage additional funds.

The FY 2001 allocation of $9.6 million is to be directed as follows:

1. **School-based initiatives**—Approximately $1.85 million is allocated for school-based programs: $1 million will be used by the Department of Education to implement health and physical education content standards in schools; $100,000 will be used to support curriculum and materials for a school resource center; and $750,000 will be provided to 16 schools over a three-year period to implement a coordinated school health program that is required to target physical activity, nutrition, and tobacco.

2. **Healthy communities initiatives**—Approximately $1 million is provided for community planning grants through a noncompetitive request for proposals (RFP) process to help community health promotion initiatives that support increased physical activity, improved nutrition, and reduced tobacco use. Key features of the grants include (1) collaboration between schools and communities, (2) a grassroots-level emphasis, and (3) a train-the-trainer model. An initial grant of up to $5,000 will provided to community groups or organizations for (a) conducting a community needs assessment and (b) developing an action plan addressing their identified priorities for support and promotion of healthy living within their community.

Upon successful completion of a sustainable community action plan that addresses one or more of the primary focus areas for HHI—physical activity promotion, nutrition, and tobacco prevention and control—participating community groups will be eligible for additional funding consideration up to $19,000 to implement their action plans.

The total funding available for community programs may be increased in FY 2002. Additionally, approximately 15 targeted interventions will be funded with funding amounts for each grant expected to range from $25,000 to $75,000. The HHI is working in collaboration with gov-

ernmental and nongovernmental agencies to integrate these efforts with other community-based health programs. For example, potential community applicants are strongly advised to create action plans that align with statewide strategies and recommendations for effective community-based activities for tobacco prevention and control, physical activity, and nutrition. Additionally, an aim of the HHI Healthy Communities Initiative is to support the development of strategies that are most likely to achieve specific environmental or system changes for the people who live and work in a defined community.

3. **Public and professional education**—Approximately $1 million is earmarked for an RFP, currently being developed for a social marketing and public awareness campaign addressing physical activity, nutrition, and tobacco use. These behaviors will be addressed both separately and together.

A funding level of $530,000 for professional education has been established, and an RFP is currently being developed. One function of the Hawaii Outcomes Institute (described in the following passage) will be that of providing professional development in the areas of assessment and evaluation, with a focus on community efforts to reduce chronic diseases.

4. **Surveillance, assessment, and evaluation**—$3.2 million will be provided to the Hawaii Outcomes Institute. The institute, which will receive $5.2 million over a two- to three-year period, is a partnership established between the Hawaii Department of Health and the University of Hawaii's John A. Burns School of Medicine to create a neutral, credible, single point of access data warehouse where data can be integrated, analyzed, and shared. Funding will be provided for three epidemiologists and one biostatistician to work with the Institute. These positions will be responsible to HHI.

Overhead Costs

Overhead costs for HHI include 15 full-time equivalent staff, which are supported with tobacco settlement funds, including physical activity and nutrition staff positions. These HHI staff members provide technical assistance to local communities, funded schools, and public and professional education initiatives.

CALIFORNIA CASE STUDY

Introduction

Similar to the situation less than a decade ago with tobacco control, today there are few large-scale nutrition and physical activity campaigns operated by states, and those that are in place have been on-line a short time. The California Nutrition Network for Healthy, Active Families (Network) is one large campaign for which cost and early outcome data are available. The Network is administered by the California Department of Health Services in partnership with the California Department of Social Services. It was chosen as a case study because it parallels the design, it targets very large population segments, and it is funded at levels close to CDC recommendations for state tobacco control programs. The example below is intended to share the experience of one state on how expenditures have been distributed among different program elements. Early evaluation results are promising but not yet conclusive.

Background

Principal federal funding for the California Nutrition Network comes from the Food Stamp Program of the U.S. Department of Agriculture (USDA). The Food Stamp Program reimburses half of all allowable cost of providing nutrition education to that portion of the audience, which is either food stamp recipients or low-income applications for the program. The funds are provided as federal financial participation that match in-kind contributions from state and local government agencies who conduct low-income targeted nutrition education. All social marketing interventions funded through the Network are intended to reach the 21% of the state's 35 million residents from households with incomes at or below 130% of the federal poverty level, the eligibility criterion for participation in the Food Stamp Program. This percentage totals over seven million persons, of which about 60% (over four million) are below the age of 18 years.

Nutrition education is an optional state administrative expense in the Food Stamp Program. Food Stamp social marketing nutrition networks grew out of a USDA initiative starting in 1995 that provided planning grants. In 2000-01, 19 states operated USDA-approved food stamp social marketing nutrition networks. While each state targets food stamp and similar low-income households, the specific population subsegments that are targeted, the intervention activities, and the federal funding levels vary. USDA guidelines for food stamp nutrition education focus heavily on dietary improvement, food security, and food safety. Therefore, the scope and nature of physical activity interventions on which USDA funds may be spent is limited, and funds may not be spent on health care delivery. In the following example, only the federal share of Network expenditures will be reported for each program category.

The expenditures reported in the following example do not include grants to California from other USDA sources such as WIC, School Meals, Food Stamps, or Cooperative Extension; or from categorical public health programs funded by the U.S. Department of Health and Human Services through the Centers for Disease Control and Prevention, the Maternal and Child Health Branch, the National Institutes of Health, Medicaid, or Medicare; nor do they include expenditures by state or local agencies or by foundations. Estimates of total expenditures of federal, state, and local expenditures for nutrition and physical activity interventions in California are not available.

History

The first state plan of the California Nutrition Network was funded by USDA in the 1996-97 federal fiscal year, and the state campaign was launched about 18 months later in August 1998. In the first year, contracts were let with 15 local public agencies; by the fifth year of operation, nearly 180 local assistance contracts were let. Federal matching funds have grown from $2.8 million in 1996-97 to $46 million in 2000-01. The total federal, state, and local effort has increased from about $5.6 million in 1996-97 to over $92 million in 2000-01. Over the years, the aims for California's low-income families with children have narrowed from overall healthy eating and exercise to just three objectives: increasing fruit and vegetable intake to five or more daily servings, increasing daily physical activity to 30 minutes in adults and 60 minutes in children, and most recently, increasing participation in the federal nutrition assistance programs, especially food stamps. Measurable impact is expected by 2003.

Evidence

There is early evidence that the California Nutrition Network is working. Although the USDA funding has limitations in its use and does not target the state's entire population, the Network's rapid growth indicates pent-up demand and a very positive response by public agencies across the state. Major nonprofit and business entities also are participating; therefore, the volume and focus of intervention activity have increased profoundly. The Network uses large-scale social marketing approaches like media, supermarket, and community-based interventions, and Network partners are encouraged to aim at least some of their intervention activities at changing policies and social and physical environments to make healthy eating and physical activity easier for low-income families in the larger community. Although the network is designed and accountable for results with low-income families with children, it would not be surprising to see positive dietary impact on Californians with higher incomes. California's fruit and vegetable emphasis is aided by the National Cancer Institute's national 5-a-Day program, which involves thousands of industry partners and provides public service media aimed at the general public.

There are promising indications of an early populationwide response to the Network interventions. A nonsignificant upward trend in fruit and vegetable intake—the principal behavioral objective of the Network—was seen in low-income adults in 1999, the most recent year for which statewide data are available (unpublished). The decline in fruit and vegetable consumption in African-Americans also stopped. While those self-reported changes occurred early in the campaign (within one year of its launch)—the findings are quite promising: Those were the groups specifically targeted by the Network; their fruit and vegetable consumption had been declining over the previous four years; and California has detected rapid population response on two previous occasions with 5-a-Day adult campaigns in media and retail channels.

Further, the changes were specific. They were seen primarily in the groups most likely to respond to promotional efforts, namely the targeted low-income segments and the highest income group. By the time of the mid-1999 survey, over 65 local agencies were working with the children and adults with the lowest income through community interventions. In addition, the Network's adult-targeted public service mass media and retail campaigns were in place.

Trends will be clearer as the results of the 2001 and 2003 state surveys and more recent national data become available, along with specific data about the reach and penetration of Network interventions. Other factors that might account for consumer change during these periods also will be taken into account.

Alignment With Recommendations for Comprehensive State Programs

The total federal financial participation approved for expenditure through the Network was $46 million in federal fiscal year (FFY) 2000-01. This budget compares to the recommendation of $165 million to $442 million for statewide tobacco control, which could be prorated as $34 million to $92 million for the 21% of California residents with incomes at or below 130% of poverty. For diet and physical activity, it is not known if a program targeted to a large subgroup is as cost-effective as one that aims for change in social norms in the entire population, nor is it known if eating and exercise interventions cost more or less on a large-scale than do those for tobacco control.

I. LEADERSHIP, PLANNING, AND COORDINATION

As cited in the CDC *Best Practices* document for state tobacco control programs, it is recommended that about 5% of a total program budget be spent on administration and management of a separate tobacco control unit charged with ensuring collaboration and coordination among public health program managers, policy makers, and other state agencies. It further recommends that a decentralized administrative system using local county and city health departments as local lead agencies be established. To operate efficiently, experience suggests that state staff are needed to ensure that there is a unified message, proper contract administration, and monitoring.

In the California Nutrition Network, about $1.3 million (or 2.3%) was spent on administration and management. This money funded about 19 full-time equivalent (FTE) state administrative staff, their travel, equipment, supplies, and indirect costs. Leadership activities included convening a large public and private steering committee and multiple advisory groups for different aspects of Network activities.

II. ENVIRONMENTAL, SYSTEMS, AND POLICY CHANGE

In tobacco control, a variety of activities are required to enforce environmental and organizational policies such as those dealing with minors' access to tobacco products and ensuring clean indoor air. The CDC *Best Practices* document for state tobacco control programs recommends a formula that included $150,000 to $300,000 for interagency coordination plus a per capita rate of $.43 to $.80, depending on number of state laws, a state's geography, and tobacco use characteristics of the state. For the entire state of California, the recommended expenditure was $14 to $26 million annually. Prorated for the 21% of the California population that falls within the Network's income eligibility, the target would be $3.1 million to $5.6 million.

State and local policy formulation in the fields of nutrition and physical activity is in a very early stage of development; thus, there are few policies to enforce. While there are recommended nutrition and physical activity policies for children in schools, such as for food sold on campus or for physical education, there is little enforcement authority and less enforcement activity. For adult environments, there are potential opportunities for the public sector to establish policies for government food services or employee work environments, and the private sector is encouraged to establish policies and direct resources toward activities that promote healthy eating and physical activity. At present that policy potential for the environments of low-income consumers is largely unrealized.

In the California Nutrition Network, a number of policy targets have been set, such as to increase campaign funding for adults and children, to establish special programs to eliminate racial, ethnic, and income associated diet and physical activity disparities, and to increase participation in available federal nutrition as-

sistance programs and help reduce food insecurity. Local contractors and sister state agencies also are encouraged to set policy objectives making affordable healthy foods more available on public property, or setting new standards or guidelines for program operations. The total separable budget for special policy projects, such as those with school officials and supermarkets, totals less than $1 million. Media advocacy to make policy makers aware of the need for new policy decisions is a thrust of both the Network's mass media and research activities.

Experience is suggesting that policy-related expenditures will grow as more is learned about the scope of the poor diet and physical inactivity problem and the limits of educational, public awareness, and promotional approaches.

III. MASS COMMUNICATIONS

The CDC *Best Practices* document for tobacco control recommends that media, or "counter-marketing," be funded at the rate of $1 to $3 per capita. For California specifically, the recommended expenditure for 1999 was $32 million to $96 million. Prorated for the 21% of California's population with incomes at or below 130% of poverty, the state target would be $6.7 million to $20 million annually. It recommended that advertising and creative firms with experience in multicultural marketing be used, and that counsel from other state agencies with media experience such as tourism or lotteries be sought. Costs were estimated based on a minimum of $100,000 per ad, and states were encouraged to share ads when possible.

The California Nutrition Network allocated slightly over $4 million for media, public relations, and placement in 2000-2001, a level that for the first time is sufficient to buy airtime rather than depend on public service in five of the state's eight largest media markets. A three-year contract was competitively bid, and the prime contractor of the winning firm develops the creative. A subcontractor with a Latino and African American staff then provides public relations, and a second subcontractor buys the media time. This level of funding supports the creative development and production of three seasonal ads for television and radio, including consumer focus groups and other consumer testing. Each is produced in English and Spanish. A small amount of outdoor advertising (billboards) and transit space (mobile billboards and wrapped busses) also is purchased in selected media markets, with an emphasis on locations near funded local projects. The media buying firm is responsible for securing maximum bonus value from media outlets in the form of on-air promotion, live-remote broadcasts tied with Network events, and public affairs programming.

For 9- to 11-year-old children, a high-quality ad was produced several years ago for sequential use in the four-year rollout of the Power Play! campaign in 11 media markets. Airtime is purchased on English and Spanish language children's programming during morning, after-school, and weekend viewing hours in the fall and again in the spring in the first year of a region's funding.

Public relation activities are usually tied with a Network or partner event, such as release of a report about California's eating or exercise practices or a policy conference. English- and Spanish-speaking spokespersons are first trained on the statewide copy points for the story, then they personalize the story. In addition, on-going communications training and public relations counsel has been made available through a public relations firm to all Network partners; its purpose is to acquaint them with techniques for localizing the issues and getting their story told. Network PR events occur about twice per year with the aim being to secure maximum media coverage across the state. A three-year communications plan in under development.

IV. COMMUNITY PROGRAMS AND COMMUNITY DEVELOPMENT

The CDC *Best Practices* document for tobacco control recommends that communities be funded with a formula that includes a base amount of $850,000 to $1,200,000 for statewide training and infrastructure, together with a per capita rate of $.70 to $2.00 annually. For California specifically, the recommended expenditure for 1999 was $23 to $65 million annually. Prorated for the 21% of the California population that falls within the Network's income eligibility, the target would be $4.8 million to $13.6 million.

The California Nutrition Network operates a less decentralized system than tobacco control does. Rather than contracting with the state's 61 local health departments, it contracts with 12 Project LEAN regional lead agencies to help coordinate activities for teens and adults and 11 Power Play! regional lead agencies for younger school-aged children. At about $100,000 per region, this smaller infrastructure totals about $2.5 million annually and is organized around the state's major media markets. A total of 67 local public agencies receive matching funds to conduct interventions based on their own needs assessments. These local agencies include 25 local health departments, four cities, four park and recreation agencies, eight Indian tribal organizations, twelve public colleges and universities, and two cooperative extensions. The amount of federal matching funds they receive varies from $5,000 to over $1 million.

In addition, 35 nonprofit and public sector organizations receive grants for faith-based, food security, or special city initiatives. These grants range in size from $15,000 to $45,000. The 49 FTE state and contract staff who support all the local contractors are funded at about $2.8 million.

In total, Network funding for community nutrition and physical activity programs and related community development totals nearly $14 million, which is close to the prorated level recommended for tobacco control.

V. PROGRAMS FOR CHILDREN AND YOUTH

In the CDC *Best Practices* document for tobacco control, it is recommended that school programs be funded through a formula that includes a base amount of $500,000 to $750,000 for statewide training and infrastructure, together with a per student rate of $4 to $6 (K-12). For California specifically, the recommended expenditure for 1999 was $25 million to $38 million. Prorated for the 40% of California's 6.5 million children aged 5-18 years, who are from households earning below 130% of poverty, the state target would be $10 million to $15.2 million annually.

Through USDA, the California Nutrition Network funds 37 low-resource school districts and county offices of education for over $12 million, with matching funds projected to range from $15,000 to over $5 million. In addition, the Network helps fund other programs such as the 5-a-Day / Power Play! campaign for fourth and fifth graders and Food on the Run for high school students to total nearly $1.9 million (additional foundation funds have been available). Total USDA matching funds dedicated solely for children and youth in school exceeded $14 million, which is close to the tobacco control target. In addition, a proportion of community development projects also serve children and youth for the most part outside school settings; thus, it is likely that Network resources helping children and youth currently exceed levels recommended for tobacco control.

It is with children and youth that the analogy with funding in tobacco control may be least applicable. Eating and exercise are complex behaviors that all children partake in many times each day, yet state data indicate that well over 75% of all children are at-risk. This statistic compares with much lower rates for tobacco use in children, a single behavior that affects a subset of young people within a more narrow age range. Furthermore, with 900 school districts and about 8,500 public schools (of which 46 percent are classified as economically "needy"—defined as below 50% of students being eligible for free/reduced price school meals) participation in the Network has barely scratched the surface. For this reason, it seems apparent that measures above and beyond those now in place in schools will be needed. Specifically, since students reflect their larger community, and time during the school day is both competitive and expensive, public health measures staged outside the school environment may be easier to conduct and possibly more cost efficient. It is also true that—as with tobacco control—efforts focusing on children alone will not succeed because adults must set an example and also create protective environments that make healthy behaviors easy for children.

VI. HEALTH CARE DELIVERY

The CDC *Best Practices* document for tobacco control recommends that specific public health programs be allocated the following base budget to develop core capacity in tobacco control: cardiovascular disease ($500,000), asthma ($1 to $1.5 million), oral health ($400,000 to $750,000), and state cancer registries ($75,000 to $300,000). It recommends a second level of funding to support more comprehensive programs that include local initiatives. For California specifically, it recommends $3.3 to $4.7 million for such programs.

For tobacco cessation, the CDC recommendations are based on an extensive literature that includes per capita costs of screening, brief counseling, and reimbursing providers for treatment programs, pharmaceuticals, and follow-up. It is noted that private insurance may cover about half the costs, and that about 10% of smokers were likely to use such services each year. The total recommended amount for California is $32 million to $120 million annually.

The California Nutrition Network provides federal matching funds for sister state categorical programs that use their own funds for allowable nutrition education to low-income Californians. The participating programs have included Cancer Detection, Child Health and Disability Prevention, Domestic Violence, Adolescent Family Life, the California Department of Education, the California Department of Food and Agriculture, and the California State Library. Most the programs use Network funds to build their core capacity or to fund special projects in nutrition and closely related topics. In 2000-2001, matching funds returned to those agencies totaled about $1.5 million.

As stated above, USDA funds may not be used for health care services; therefore, there is no Network experience paying for medical nutrition treatment or physical therapy services. However, a new study of the health care costs of obesity in California adults is underway and will be reported shortly.

SURVEILLANCE, EPIDEMIOLOGY, AND RESEARCH

The CDC *Best Practices* document for tobacco control recommends as standard practice that about 10% of a total program budget (excluding administration) be dedicated to surveillance and evaluation. Those activities might strengthen the statewide program or the capacity of local programs. They include surveys, research, and evaluation conducted by the state health department, by universities or private research firms, or by local projects. For California specifically, the recommendation is for $14 million to $38 million annually.

The California Nutrition Network spent about $1.5 million on surveys and applied research in 2000-2001. The annualized budget supports partial funding for the following: the state's three biennial eating and exercise surveys for adults, teens, and older children (grant funds are also available for this purpose); questions on two large omnibus state surveys; formative research using focus groups, surveys, and key informant interviews; contracted evaluation specialists for interventions in several channels; and special policy studies. Including the staff of five FTE's and excluding evaluation conducted by local projects, expenditures for research and evaluation are estimated at about $2.1 million in 2000-2001, or about 4% of the annual budget.

An additional $2 million is made available annually from state funds through the Cancer Research Program to support a variety of intramural diet and behavior change prevention projects, including a university-based social marketing center, intervention projects, and several policy analyses.

REFERENCES AND RESOURCES

1. Centers for Disease Control and Prevention, *Best Practices for Comprehensive Tobacco Control Programs—August 1999.* Atlanta, GA: US Department of Health and Human Services, Center for Disease Control and Prevention, National Center for Chronic Disease Prevention and Health Promotions, Office on Smoking and Health, August 1999.

2. California Department of Health Services, *California Dietary Practices Survey, Overall Trends in Healthy Eating Among Adults, 1989-1997, A Call to Action, Part 2.* Sacramento, CA 1999.

APPENDIX B

Linking the Guidelines to the Essential Public Health Services

The *Guidelines for Comprehensive Programs to Promote Healthy Eating and Physical Activity* is an operational framework for delivering the Essential Public Health Services for nutrition and physical activity. The descriptive activities are as follows:

• **Leadership, planning/management, and coordination**—Create a culture for public health competence; develop supportive policies and guidelines; generate fiscal support for nutrition and physical activity programs; provide essential and extended staffing and resources; assess the quality, acceptability, and accessibility of nutrition and physical activity programs.

• **Environmental, systems, and policy change**—Use social marketing approaches to define needs and diagnose problems; create awareness with stakeholders and the public about the contribution of policy and environment to health; mobilize support for programs through coalitions and partnerships including nontraditional partners; develop policies designed to change norms; enforce legislative and policy initiatives; evaluate population-wide program effects.

• **Mass communication**—Make use of the media to inform and to create awareness and discussion of nutrition and physical activity issues; highlight priority needs; identify innovative solutions and research findings; pretest messages and concepts with constituents; and evaluate media effects.

• **Community programs and community development**—Mobilize and empower the community for action; develop coalitions and partnerships around important nutrition and physical activity issues; assist communities to assess needs and to develop plans to address priority problems; conduct sensitive and appropriate interventions; ensure that program outcomes are measured.

• **Programs for children and youth**—Assess the health status and practices of youth; develop healthful school policies and guidelines; mobilize teachers, parents, and the community for action related to nutrition and physical activity; enforce laws, guidelines, and policies; evaluate curricula and programs for quality and effectiveness.

• **Health care delivery**—Develop effective protocols for prevention and treatment; link those in need to appropriate services; educate clients about healthful practices.

• **Surveillance, epidemiology, and research**—Conduct community assessments and audits; investigate causal associations with inactivity and poor diet; evaluate program effects; test innovative programs in community settings.